The Vibrant Air Fryer Cooking Guide

Easy And Healthy Air Fryer Recipes For Beginners

Ellie Sloan

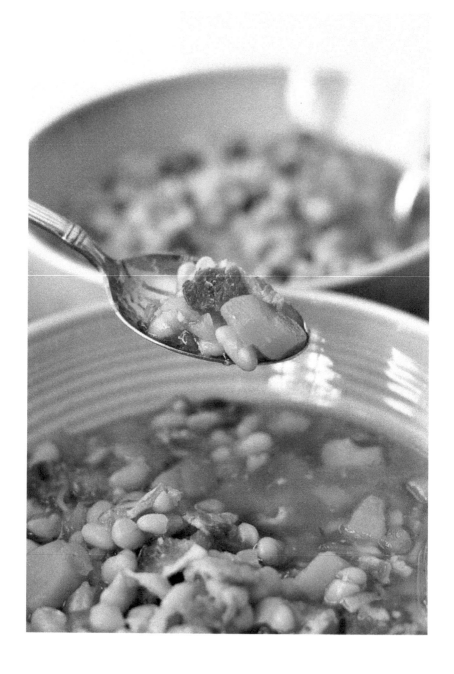

Table of contents

Cheese and Ham Patties

Preparation Time: 10 minutes

Cooking Time: 10 minutes

Servings: 4

Ingredients:

- 1 puff pastry sheet
- 4 handfuls mozzarella cheese, grated
- 4 tsp.s mustard
- 8 ham slices, chopped

Directions:

1. Spread out puff pastry on a clean surface and cut it in 12 squares.
2. Divide cheese, ham, and mustard on half of them, top with the other halves, and seal the edges.
3. Place all the patties in your Air Fryer's basket and cook at 370°F for 10 minutes.

4. Divide the patties between plates and serve.

Nutrition:

Calories 212

Fat 12g

Carbs 14g

Protein 8g

Buttered Scallops

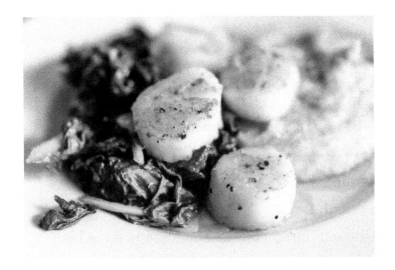

Preparation Time: 15 minutes

Cooking Time: 4 minutes

Servings: 2

Ingredients:

- ¾ lb. sea scallops, cleaned and patted very dry
- 1 tbsp. butter, melted
- ½ tbsp. fresh thyme, minced

- Salt and black pepper, as required

Directions:

1. Preheat the Air Fryer to 390°F and grease an Air Fryer basket.
2. Mix scallops, butter, thyme, salt, and black pepper in a bowl.
3. Arrange scallops in the Air Fryer basket and cook for about 4 minutes.
4. Dish out the scallops in a platter and serve hot.

Nutrition:

Calories 202,

Fat 7.1g

Carbs 4.4g

Protein 28.7g

Butter Trout

Preparation Time: 5 minutes

Cooking Time: 20 minutes

Servings: 4

Ingredients:

- trout fillets; boneless
- Juice of 1 lime
- 1 tbsp. parsley; chopped.
- tbsp. butter; melted
- Salt and black pepper to taste.

Directions:

1. Mix the fish fillets with the melted butter, salt and pepper, rub gently, put the fish in your Air Fryer's basket and cook at 390°F for 6 minutes on each side.
2. Divide between plates and serve with lime juice drizzled on top and with parsley sprinkled at the end.

Nutrition:

Calories 221

Fat 11g

Carbs 6g

Protein 9g

Pesto Almond Salmon

Preparation Time: 5 minutes

Cooking Time: 15 minutes

Servings: 4

Ingredients:

- 2 1 ½-inch-thick salmon fillets: about 4 oz. each
- ¼ cup sliced almonds, roughly chopped
- ¼ cup pesto
- tbsp. unsalted butter; melted.

Directions:

1. In a small bowl, mix pesto and almonds. Set aside. Place fillets into a 6-inch round baking dish
2. Brush each fillet with butter and place half of the pesto mixture on the top of each fillet. Place dish into the Air Fryer basket. Set the temperature to 390°F and set the timer for 12 minutes

3. Salmon will easily flake when fully cooked and reach an internal temperature of at least 145°F. Serve warm.

Nutrition:

Calories 433

Fat 34.0g

Protein 23.3g

Carbs 6.1g

Garlic Lemon Shrimp

Preparation Time: 5 minutes

Cooking Time: 10 minutes

Servings: 4

Ingredients:

- 8 oz. medium shelled and deveined shrimp
- 1 medium lemon.
- 2 tbsp. unsalted butter; melted.
- ½ tsp. minced garlic
- ½ tsp. Old Bay seasoning

Directions:

1. Zest lemon and then cut in half. Place shrimp in a large bowl and squeeze juice from ½ lemon on top of them.
2. Add lemon zest to bowl along with remaining ingredients. Toss shrimp until fully coated
3. Pour bowl contents into 6-inch round baking dish. Place into the Air Fryer basket.

4. Adjust the temperature to 400°F and set the timer for 6 minutes. Shrimp will be bright pink when fully cooked. Serve warm with pan sauce.

Nutrition:

Calories 190

Fat 11.8g

Protein 16.4g

Carbs 2.9g

Air-Fried Crab Sticks

Preparation Time: 5 minutes

Cooking Time: 10 minutes

Servings: 4

Ingredients:

- Crab sticks: 1 package
- Cooking oil spray: as needed

Directions:

1. Take each of the sticks out of the package and unroll until flat. Tear the sheets into thirds.
2. Arrange them on a plate and lightly spritz using cooking spray. Set the timer for 10 minutes at 360°F.
3. Note: If you shred the crab meat; you can cut the time in half, but they will also easily fall through the holes in the basket.

Nutrition:

Calories 220

Fat 13g

Carbs 11g

Protein 23g

E-Z Catfish

Preparation Time: 5 minutes

Cooking Time: 25 minutes

Servings: 3

Ingredients:

- Olive oil: 1 tbsp.
- Seasoned fish fry: .25 cup
- Catfish fillets: 4

Directions:

1. Prepare the fryer to 400°F.
2. First, wash the fish, and dry with a paper towel.
3. Dump the seasoning into a large zip-type baggie. Add the fish and shake to cover each fillet. Spray with a spritz of cooking oil spray. Add to the basket.
4. Set the timer for ten minutes. Flip, and reset the timer for ten more minutes. Flip once more and cook for two to three minutes.

5. Once it reaches the desired crispiness, transfer to a plate to serve.

Nutrition:

Calories 290

Carbs 14g

Fat 16g

Protein 30g

Fish Nuggets

Preparation Time: 5 minutes

Cooking Time: 20 minutes

Servings: 4

Ingredients:

- Cod fillet: 1 lb.
- Eggs: 3
- Olive oil: 4 tbsp.
- Almond flour: 1 cup
- Gluten-free breadcrumbs: 1 cup

Directions:

1. Fix the temperature of the Air Fryer at 390°F.
2. Cut the cod into nuggets.
3. Prepare three dishes. Beat the eggs in one. Combine the oil and breadcrumbs in another. The last one will be almond flour.

4. Cover each of the nuggets using the flour, a dip in the eggs, and the breadcrumbs.

5. Arrange the prepared nuggets in the basket and set the timer for 20 minutes. Serve.

Nutrition:

Calories 220

Carbs 10g

Fat 12g

Protein 23g

Grilled Shrimp

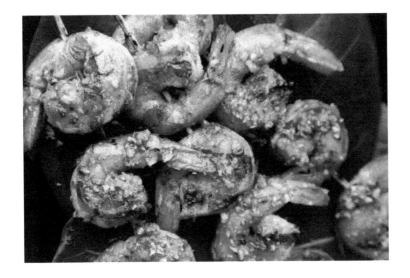

Preparation Time: 5 minutes

Cooking Time: 10 minutes

Servings: 4

Ingredients:

- Medium shrimp/prawns: 8
- Melted butter: 1 tbsp.
- Rosemary: 1 sprig

- Pepper and salt: as desired
- Minced garlic cloves: 3

Directions:

1. Combine all of the fixings in a mixing bowl. Toss well and arrange in the fryer basket.
2. Set the timer for 7 minutes: 356°F and serve.

Nutrition:

Calories 180

Fat 10g

Carbs 2g

Protein 15g

Honey & Sriracha Tossed Calamari

Preparation Time: 10 minutes

Cooking Time: 20 minutes

Servings: 2

Ingredients:

- Calamari tubes - tentacles if you prefer: .5 lb.
- Club soda: 1 cup
- Flour: 1 cup
- Salt - red pepper & black pepper: 2 dashes each
- Honey: .5 cup+ 1-2 tbsp. Sriracha

Directions:

1. Fully rinse the calamari and blot it dry using a bunch of paper towels. Slice into rings: .25-inch wide). Toss the rings into a bowl. Pour in the club soda and stir until all are submerged. Wait for about 10 minutes.
2. Sift the salt, flour, red & black pepper. Set aside for now.

3. Dredge the calamari into the flour mixture and set on a platter until ready to fry.
4. Spritz the basket of the Air Fryer with a small amount of cooking oil spray. Arrange the calamari in the basket, careful not to crowd it too much.
5. Set the temperature at 375°F and the timer for 11 minutes.
6. Shake the basket twice during the cooking process, loosening any rings that may stick.
7. Remove from the basket, toss with the sauce, and return to the fryer for two more minutes.
8. Serve with additional sauce as desired.
9. Make the sauce by combining honey, and sriracha, in a small bowl, mix until fully combined.

Nutrition:

Calories 210

Fat 12g

Carbs 5g

Protein 19g

Salmon Croquettes

Preparation Time: 5 minutes

Cooking Time: 10 minutes

Servings: 4

Ingredients:

- Red salmon: 1 lb. can
- Breadcrumbs: 1 cup
- Vegetable oil: .33 cup
- Chopped parsley: half of 1 bunch
- Eggs: 2

Directions:

1. Set the Air Fryer at 392°F.
2. Drain and mash the salmon. Whisk and add the eggs and parsley.
3. In another dish, mix the breadcrumbs and oil.
4. Prepare 16 croquettes using the breadcrumb mixture.
5. Arrange in the preheated fryer basket for 7 minutes.

6. Serve.

Nutrition:

Calories 240

Fat 16g

Carbs 7g

Protein 30g

Spicy Cod

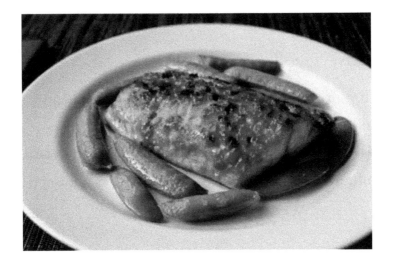

Preparation Time: 5 minutes

Cooking Time: 10 minutes

Servings: 4

Ingredients:

- 4 cod fillets; boneless
- 2 tbsp. assorted chili peppers
- 1 lemon; sliced

- Juice of 1 lemon
- Salt and black pepper to taste

Directions:

1. In your Air Fryer, mix the cod with the chili pepper, lemon juice, salt and pepper
2. Arrange the lemon slices on top and cook at 360°F for 10 minutes. Divide the fillets between plates and serve.

Nutrition:

Calories 250

Fat 13g

Carbs 13g

Protein 29g

Air Fried Lobster Tails

Preparation Time: 5 minutes

Cooking Time: 10 minutes

Servings: 2

Ingredients:

- 2 tbsp. unsalted butter, melted
- 1 tbsp. minced garlic
- 1 tsp. salt
- 1 tbsp. minced fresh chives
- 2 (4- to 6 oz.) frozen lobster tails

Directions:

1. In a bowl, put the butter, garlic, salt, and chives then mix.
2. Butterfly the lobster tail: Starting at the meaty end of the tail, use kitchen shears to cut down the center of the top shell. Stop when you reach the fanned, wide part of the tail. Carefully spread apart the meat and the shell along the cut line, but keep the meat attached where it connects to the

wide part of the tail. Use your hand to gently disconnect the meat from the bottom of the shell. Lift the meat up and out of the shell (keeping it attached at the wide end). Close the shell under the meat, so the meat rests on top of the shell.

3. Place the lobster in the Air Fryer basket and generously brush the butter mixture over the meat.

4. Set the temperature of your Air Fryer to 380°F. Set the timer and steam for 4 minutes.

5. Open the Air Fryer and rotate the lobster tails. Brush them with more of the butter mixture. Reset the timer and steam for 4 minutes more. The lobster is done when the meat is opaque.

Nutrition:

Calories 255

Fat 13g

Carbs 2g

Protein 32g

Air Fryer Salmon

Preparation Time: 5 minutes

Cooking Time: 10 minutes

Servings: 2

Ingredients:

- ½ tsp. salt
- ½ tsp. garlic powder
- ½ tsp. smoked paprika
- Salmon

Directions:

1. Mix spices together and sprinkle onto salmon. Place seasoned salmon into the Air Fryer.
2. Close crisping lid. Set temperature to 400°F, and set time to 10 minutes.

Nutrition:

Calories 185

Fat 11g

Carbs 12g

Protein21g

Simple Scallops

Preparation Time: 5 minutes

Cooking Time: 5 minutes

Servings: 4

Ingredients:

- 12 medium sea scallops
- 1 tsp. fine sea salt
- ground black pepper as desired
- Fresh thyme leaves, for garnish (optional)

Directions:

1. Grease the Air Fryer basket with avocado oil. Preheat the Air Fryer to 390°F. Rinse the scallops and pat completely dry. Spray avocado oil on the scallops and season them with the salt and pepper.
2. Place them in the Air Fryer basket, spacing them apart (if you're using a smaller Air Fryer, work in batches if necessary). Flip the scallops after cooking for 2 minutes,

and cook for another 2 minutes, or until cooked through and no longer translucent. Garnish with ground black pepper and thyme leaves, if desired. Best served fresh.

Nutrition:

Calories 170

Fat 11g

Carbs 8g

Protein 17g

3-Ingredient Air Fryer Catfish

Preparation Time: 5 minutes

Cooking Time: 15 minutes

Servings: 4

Ingredients:

- 1 tbsp. chopped parsley
- 1 tbsp. olive oil
- ¼ C. seasoned fish fry
- 4 catfish fillets

Directions:

1. Ensure your Air Fryer is preheated to 400°F.
2. Rinse off catfish fillets and pat dry. Add fish fry seasoning to Ziploc baggie, then catfish. Shake bag and ensure fish gets well coated. Spray each fillet with olive oil. Add fillets to Air Fryer basket.

3. Set temperature to 400°F, and set time to 10 minutes. Cook 10 minutes. Then flip and cook another 2-3 minutes.

Nutrition:

Calories 208

Fat 5g

Carbs 5g

Protein 17g

Pecan-Crusted Catfish

Preparation Time: 5 minutes

Cooking Time: 12 minutes

Servings: 4

Ingredients:

- ½ cup pecan meal
- 1 tsp. fine sea salt
- ¼ tsp. ground black pepper
- 4 (4 oz.) catfish fillets
- For garnish (optional) Fresh oregano

Directions:

1. Grease the Air Fryer basket with avocado oil. Preheat the Air Fryer to 375°F. In a large bowl, mix the pecan meal, salt, and pepper. One at a time, dredge the catfish fillets in the mixture, coating them well. Use your hands to press the pecan meal into the fillets. Spray the fish with avocado oil and place them in the Air Fryer basket.

2. Cook the coated catfish for 12 minutes, or until it flakes easily and is no longer translucent in the center, flipping halfway through. Garnish with oregano sprigs and pecan halves, if desired.

Nutrition:

Calories 162

Fat 11g

Carbs 1g

Protein 17g

Flying Fish

Preparation Time: 5 minutes

Cooking Time: 12 minutes

Servings: 4

Ingredients:

- Tbsp. Oil
- 3–4 oz Breadcrumbs
- 1 Whisked Whole Egg in a Saucer/Soup Plate
- 4 Fresh Fish Fillets
- Fresh Lemon (For serving)

Directions:

1. Warm up the Air Fryer to 350°F. Mix the crumbs and oil until it looks nice and loose. Dip the fish in the egg and coat lightly, then move on to the crumbs. Make sure the fillet is covered evenly.

2. Cook in the Air Fryer basket for roughly 12 minutes – depending on the size of the fillets you are using. Serve with fresh lemon & chips to complete the duo.

Nutrition:

Calories 180

Fat 12g

Carbs 9g

Protein 19g

Air Fryer Fish Tacos

Preparation Time: 5 minutes

Cooking Time: 15 minutes

Servings: 4

Ingredients:

- 1 lb. cod
- 1 tbsp. cumin
- ½ tbsp. chili powder
- 1 ½ C. coconut flour
- 10 oz. Mexican beer
- 2 eggs

Directions:

1. Whisk beer and eggs together. Whisk flour, pepper, salt, cumin, and chili powder together. Slice cod into large pieces and coat in egg mixture then flour mixture.
2. Spray bottom of your Air Fryer basket with olive oil and add coated codpieces. Cook 15 minutes at 375°F.

43

3. Serve on lettuce leaves topped with homemade salsa.

Nutrition:

Calories 178

Fat 10g

Carbs 61g

Protein 19g

Bacon Wrapped Scallops

Preparation Time: 5 minutes

Cooking Time: 5 minutes

Servings: 4

Ingredients:

- 1 tsp. paprika
- 1 tsp. lemon pepper
- 5 slices of center-cut bacon
- 20 raw sea scallops

Directions:

1. Rinse and drain scallops, placing on paper towels to soak up excess moisture. Cut slices of bacon into 4 pieces. With a piece of bacon, wrap each scallop, then using toothpicks to secure. Sprinkle wrapped scallops with paprika and lemon pepper.
2. Spray Air Fryer basket with olive oil and add scallops.

3. Cook 5-6 minutes at 400°F, making sure to flip halfway through.

Nutrition:

Calories 389

Fat17g

Carbs 63g

Protein 21g

Quick Fried Catfish

Preparation Time: 5 minutes

Cooking Time: 15 minutes

Servings: 4

Ingredients:

- 3/4 cups Original Bisquick™ mix
- 1/2 cup yellow cornmeal
- 1 tbsp. seafood seasoning
- 4 catfish fillets (4-6 oz. each)
- 1/2 cup ranch dressing

Directions:

1. In a bowl mix the Bisquick mix, cornmeal, and seafood seasoning together. Pat the filets dry, then brush them with ranch dressing. Press the filets into the Bisquick mix on both sides until the filet is evenly coated.
2. Cook in your Air Fryer at 360°For 15 minutes, flip the filets halfway through. Serve.

Nutrition:

Calories 372

Fat 16g

Carbs 14g

Protein 28g

Air-Fried Herbed Shrimp

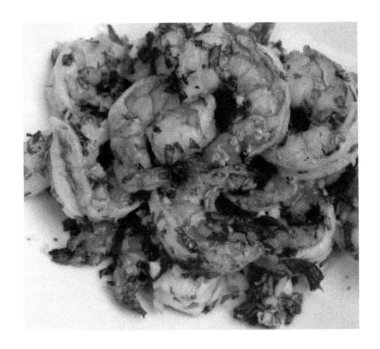

Preparation Time: 2 minutes

Cooking Time: 5 minutes

Servings: 4

Ingredients:

- One ¼ lb. shrimp, peeled and deveined

- ½ tsp. paprika
- One tbsp. olive oil
- ¼ cayenne pepper
- ½ tsp. Old Bay seasoning

Directions:

1. Preheat Air Fryer to 400°F. Mix all the ingredients in a bowl. Place the seasoned shrimp into the Air Fryer basket and cook for 5-minutes.

Nutrition:

Calories 300

Fat 9.3g

Carbs 8.2g

Protein 14.6g

Wild Caught Salmon

Preparation Time: 5 minutes

Cooking Time: 12 minutes

Servings: 2

Ingredients:

- 2 salmon fillets, wild-caught, each about 1 ½ inch thick
- 1 tsp. ground black pepper
- 2 tsp. paprika
- 1 tsp. salt
- 2 tsp. olive oil

Directions:

1. Switch on the air fryer, insert fryer basket, grease it with olive oil, then shut with its lid, set the fryer at 390°F and preheat for 5 minutes. Meanwhile, rub each salmon fillet with oil and then season with black pepper, paprika, and salt.

2. Open the fryer, add seasoned salmon in it, close with its lid and cook for 7 minutes until nicely golden and cooked, flipping the fillets halfway through the frying.when air fryer beeps, open its lid, transfer salmon onto a serving plate and serve.

Nutrition:

Calories 288

Carbs 1.4g

Fat 18.9g

Protein 28.3g

Crispy Keto Pork Bites

Preparation Time: 5 minutes

Cooking Time: 25 minutes

Servings: 2

Ingredients:

- 1 medium onion
- ½ lb. pork belly
- tbsp. coconut cream
- 1 tbsp. butter
- Salt & pepper, to taste

Directions:

1. Slice the pork belly into even and thin strips
2. The onion has to be diced.
3. Transfer all the ingredients into a mixing bowl and allow it to marinate in the fridge for the next two hours.
4. Fix the temperature to 350°F and preheat the Air Fryer for 5 minutes.

5. Keep the pork strips inside the Air Fryer and let it cook for 25 minutes at a temperature of 350°F.
6. Enjoy!

Nutrition:

Calories 448

Fat 42g

Carbs 2g

Protein 20g

Keto Air Bread

Preparation Time: 10 minutes

Cooking Time: 25 minutes

Serving: 19

Ingredients:

- 1 cup almond flour
- ¼ sea salt
- 1 tsp. baking powder
- ¼ cup butter
- 3 eggs

Directions:

1. Crack the eggs into a bowl then using a hand blender mix them up. Melt the butter at room temperature. Take the melted butter and add it to the egg mixture. Add the salt, baking powder and almond flour to egg mixture and knead the dough.

2. Cover the prepared dough with a towel for 10-minutes to rest. Meanwhile, preheat your Air Fryer to 360°F.
3. Place the prepared dough in the Air Fryer tin and cook the bread for 10-minutes. Then reduce the heat to 350°F and cook the bread for additional 15-minutes you can use a toothpick to check to make sure the bread is cooked.
4. Transfer the bread to a wooden board to allow it to chill. Once the bread has chilled, then slice and serve it.

Nutrition:

Calories 40

Fat 3.9g

Carbs 0.5g

Protein 1.2g

Herbed Breakfast Eggs

Preparation Time: 10 minutes

Cooking Time: 17 minutes

Serving: 2

Ingredients:

- 4 eggs
- 1 tsp. oregano
- 1 tsp. parsley, dried
- ½ tsp. sea salt
- 1 tbsp. chives, chopped
- 1 tbsp. cream
- 1 tsp. paprika

Directions:

1. Place the eggs in the Air Fryer basket and cook them for 17-minutes at 320°F. Meanwhile, combine the parsley, oregano, cream, and salt in shallow bowl.

2. Chop the chives and add them to cream mixture. When the eggs are cooked, place them in cold water and allow them to chill. After this, peel the eggs and cut them into halves.

3. Remove the egg yolks and add yolks to cream mixture and mash to blend well with a fork. Then fill the egg whites with the cream-egg yolk mixture. Serve immediately.

Nutrition:

Calories 136

Fat 9.3g

Carbs 2.1g

Protein 11.4g

Eggs in Zucchini Nests

Preparation Time: 10 minutes

Cooking Time: 7 minutes

Serving: 2

Ingredients:

- 4 tsp.s butter
- ½ tsp. paprika
- ½ tsp. black pepper
- ¼ tsp. sea salt
- 4 oz. cheddar cheese, shredded
- 4 eggs
- 8 oz. zucchini, grated

Directions:

1. Grate the zucchini and place the butter in ramekins. Add the grated zucchini in ramekins in the shape of nests.

Sprinkle the zucchini nests with salt, pepper, and paprika. Beat the eggs and pour over zucchini nests.

2. Top egg mixture with shredded cheddar cheese. Preheat the Air Fryer basket at 360°F and cook the dish for 7-minutes. When the zucchini nests are cooked, chill them for 3 minutes and serve them in the ramekins.

Nutrition:

Calories 221

Fat 17.7g

Carbs 2.9g

Protein 13.4g

Breakfast Liver Pate

Preparation Time: 5 minutes

Cooking Time: 10 minutes

Serving: 7

Ingredients:

- 1 lb. chicken liver
- 1 tsp. salt
- ½ tsp. cilantro, dried
- 1 yellow onion, diced
- 1 tsp. ground black pepper
- 1 cup water
- 4 tbsp. butter

Directions:

1. Chop the chicken liver roughly and place it in the Air Fryer basket tray. Add water to Air Fryer basket tray and add diced onion. Preheat your Air Fryer to 360°F and cook

61

chicken liver for 10-minutes. Dry out the chicken liver when it is finished cooking.

2. Transfer the chicken liver to blender, add butter, ground black pepper and dried cilantro and blend. Once you get a pate texture, transfer to liver pate bowl and serve immediately or keep in the fridge for later.

Nutrition:

Calories 173

Fat 10.8g

Carbs 2.2g

Protein 16.1g

Bread-Free Breakfast Sandwich

Preparation Time: 10 minutes

Cooking Time: 10 minutes

Serving: 2

Ingredients:

- 6 oz. ground chicken
- 2 slices of cheddar cheese
- 2 lettuce leaves
- 1 tbsp. dill, dried
- ½ tsp. sea salt
- 1 egg
- 1 tsp. cayenne pepper
- 1 tsp. tomato puree

Directions:

1. Combine the ground chicken with the pepper and sea salt. Add the dried dill and stir. Beat the egg into the

ground chicken mixture. Make 2 medium-sized burgers from the ground chicken mixture.

2. Preheat your Air Fryer to 380°F. Spray the Air Fryer basket tray with olive oil and place the ground chicken burgers inside of it. Cook the chicken burgers for 10-minutes Flip over burgers and cook for an additional 6-minutes. When the burgers are cooked, transfer them to the lettuce leaves.

3. Sprinkle the top of them with tomato puree and with a slice of cheddar cheese. Serve immediately!

Nutrition:

Calories 324

Fat 19.2g

Carbs 2.3g

Protein 34.8g

Egg Butter

Preparation Time: 5 minutes

Cooking Time: 17 minutes

Serving: 2

Ingredients:

- 4 eggs
- 4 tbsp. butter
- 1 tsp. salt

Directions:

1. Cover the Air Fryer basket with foil and place the eggs there. Transfer the Air Fryer basket into the Air Fryer and cook the eggs for 17 minutes at 320°F.
2. When the time is over, remove the eggs from the Air Fryer basket and put them in cold water to chill them. After this, peel the eggs and chop them up finely. Combine the chopped eggs with butter and add salt.

3. Mix it until you get the spread texture. Serve the egg butter with the keto almond bread.

Nutrition:

Calories 164

Fat 8.5g

Carbs 2.67g

Protein 3g

Awesome Lemon Bell Peppers

Preparation Time: 10 minutes

Cooking Time: 5 minutes

Serving: 4

Ingredients:

- 4 bell peppers
- 1 tsp. olive oil
- 1 tbsp. lemon juice
- 1/4 tsp. garlic, minced
- 1 tsp. parsley, chopped
- 1 pinch sea salt
- Pinch of pepper

Directions:

1. Preheat your Air Fryer to 390°F
2. Add bell pepper in the Air Fryer. Drizzle with it with the olive oil and air fry for 5 minutes

3. Take a serving plate and transfer it. Take a small bowl and add garlic, parsley, lemon juice, salt, and pepper
4. Mix them well and Drizzle with the mixture over the peppers. Serve and enjoy!

Nutrition:

Calories 59

Fat 4g

Carbs 6g

Protein 2g

Creamy Potatoes

Preparation Time: 10 minutes

Cooking Time: 20 minutes

Servings: 2

Ingredients:

- ¾ lb. potatoes, peeled and cubed
- 1 tbsp. olive oil
- Salt and black pepper, to taste
- ½ tbsp. hot paprika
- ½ cup Greek yogurt

Directions:

1. Place potatoes in a bowl, pour water to cover, and leave aside for 10 minutes. Drain, pat dry, then transfer to another bowl.
2. Add salt, pepper, paprika, and half of the oil to the potatoes and mix.

3. Put potatoes in the Air Fryer basket and cook at 360°F for 20 minutes.
4. In a bowl, mix yogurt with salt, pepper, and the rest of the oil and whisk.
5. Divide potatoes onto plates, drizzle with yogurt dressing, mix, and serve.

Nutrition:

Calories 170

Fat 3g

Carb: 2g

Protein 5g

Green Beans and Cherry Tomatoes

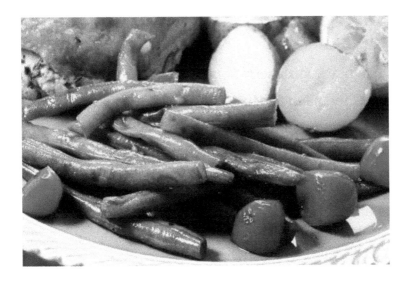

Preparation Time: 10 minutes

Cooking Time: 15 minutes

Servings: 2

Ingredients:

- 8 oz. cherry tomatoes
- 8 oz. green beans
- 1 tbsp. olive oil

- Salt and black pepper, to taste

Directions:

1. In a bowl, mix cherry tomatoes with green beans, olive oil, salt, and pepper. Mix.
2. Cook in the Air Fryer at 400°F for 15 minutes. Shake once. Serve.

Nutrition:

Calories 162

Fat 6g

Carb: 8g

Protein 9g

Crispy Brussels Sprouts and Potatoes

Preparation Time: 10 minutes

Cooking Time: 8 minutes

Servings: 2

Ingredients:

- ¾ lb. brussels sprouts, washed and trimmed
- ½ cup new potatoes, chopped
- 2 tsp.s bread crumbs
- Salt and black pepper, to taste
- 2 tsp.s butter

Directions:

1. In a bowl, add Brussels sprouts, potatoes, bread crumbs, salt, pepper, and butter. Mix well.
2. Place in the Air Fryer and cook at 400°F for 8 minutes. Serve.

Nutrition:

Calories 152

Fat 3g

Carb: 7g

Protein 4g

Herbed Tomatoes

Preparation Time: 10 minutes

Cooking Time: 15 minutes

Servings: 2

Ingredients:

- 2 big tomatoes, halved and insides scooped out
- Salt and black pepper, to taste
- ½ tbsp. olive oil
- 1 clove garlic, minced
- ¼ tsp. thyme, chopped

Directions:

1. In the Air Fryer, mix tomatoes with thyme, garlic, oil, salt, and pepper.
2. Mix and cook at 390°F for 15 minutes. Serve.

Nutrition:

Calories 112

Fat 1g

Carb: 4g

Protein 4g

Air Fried Leeks

Preparation Time: 10 minutes

Cooking Time: 7 minutes

Servings: 2

Ingredients:

- 2 leeks, washed, ends cut, and halved
- Salt and black pepper, to taste
- ½ tbsp. butter, melted
- ½ tbsp. lemon juice

Directions:

1. Rub leeks with melted butter and season with salt and pepper.
2. Lay it inside the Air Fryer and cook at 350F for 7 minutes.
3. Arrange on a platter. Drizzle with lemon juice and serve.

Nutrition:

Calories 100

Fat 4g

Carb: 6g

Protein 2g

Crispy Broccoli

Preparation Time: 10 minutes

Cooking Time: 10 minutes

Servings: 4

Ingredients:

- 1 large head fresh broccoli
- 2 tsp.s olive oil
- tbsp. lemon juice

Directions:

1. Rinse the broccoli and pat dry. Cut off the florets and separate them. You can also use the broccoli stems too; cut them into 1″ chunks and peel them.
2. Toss the broccoli, olive oil, and lemon juice in a large bowl until coated.
3. Roast the broccoli in the Air Fryer at 365°F, in batches, for 10 to 14 minutes or until the broccoli is crisp-tender and

slightly brown around the edges. Repeat with the remaining broccoli. Serve immediately.

Nutrition:

Calories 63

Fat 2g

Carbs 10g

Protein 4g

Garlic-Roasted Bell Peppers

Preparation Time: 5 minutes

Cooking Time: 20 minutes

Servings: 4

Ingredients:

- 4 bell peppers, any colors, stemmed, seeded, membranes removed, and cut into fourths
- 1 tsp. olive oil
- 4 garlic cloves, minced
- ½ tsp. dried thyme

Directions:

1. Put the peppers in the basket of the Air Fryer and drizzle with olive oil. Toss gently. Roast for 15 minutes at 365°F.
2. Sprinkle with the garlic and thyme. Roast for 3 to 5 minutes more, or until tender. Serve immediately.

Nutrition:

Calories 36

Fat 1g

Carbs 5g

Protein 1g

Asparagus with Garlic

Preparation Time: 5 minutes

Cooking Time: 10 minutes

Servings: 4

Ingredients:

- 1-lb. asparagus, rinsed, ends snapped off where they naturally break
- 2 tsp.s olive oil
- 3 garlic cloves, minced
- 2 tbsp. balsamic vinegar
- ½ tsp. dried thyme

Directions:

1. In a huge bowl, mix the asparagus with olive oil. -Transfer to the Air Fryer basket.
2. Sprinkle with garlic. Roast for 4 to 5 minutes at 375°F for crisp-tender or for 8 to 11 minutes for asparagus that is crisp on the outside and tender on the inside.

3. Drizzle with the balsamic vinegar and sprinkle with the thyme leaves. Serve immediately.

Nutrition:

Calories 41

Fat 1g

Carbs 6g

Protein 3g

Instant Lamb Steak with Apples and Pears

Preparation Time: 10 minutes

Cooking Time: 1 hour

Servings: 3

Ingredients:

- 2 lamb steaks
- 3 Arkansas Black apples, sliced
- 2 pears, sliced
- 3 tbsp. melted butter
- 4 kale leaves
- 2 tbsp. apple cider
- ½ tsp. ground black pepper
- 1 medium white onion, cut into 8 wedges
- ½ tsp. ground allspice
- 1 tsp. black pepper

Directions:

1. In a skillet, melt the butter and Put the Air Fryer to sauté mode and spoon the melted butter.
2. Add in the lamb steaks and sauté for around 20 minutes.
3. Transfer the lamb to a plate.
4. Add in the onion, apples and pears in the Air Fryer and allow them to sauté for 10 minutes until the apples are somewhat browned and caramelized.
5. Add in the lamb and pour the apple cider on top. Combine all the ingredients (except kale) and close the lid to cook for 20-30 minutes on a HIGH pressure.
6. Portion the lamb into two plates. Serve the lamb with the apples and fresh kale.

Nutrition:

Calories 379

Fat 79g

Carbs 279g

Protein 68g

Adobo Chicken

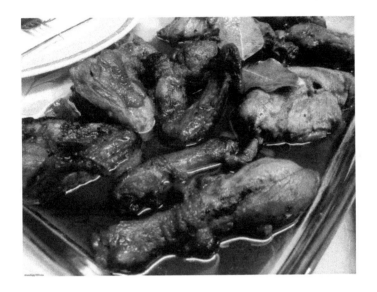

Preparation Time: 5 minutes

Cooking Time: 30 minutes

Servings: 6

Ingredients:

- 2 lbs. Chicken, Boneless
- 1 Tbsp. Turmeric
- 1 Tbsp. Garlic

- 4 Tomatoes, Chopped
- 7 Oz. Green Chilies
- ½ Cup Water

Directions:

1. Put your chicken into your Air Fryer and then seasoning it. Add in your chilies and tomatoes.
2. Empty your water in, and then cook for twenty-five minutes before using a quick release. Serve on its own or over rice.

Nutrition:

Calories 342

Fat 19g

Carbs 2g

Protein 32g

Tomato & Feta Shrimp

Preparation Time: 5 minutes

Cooking Time: 25 minutes

Servings: 6

Ingredients:

- 1 ½ Cups Onion, Chopped
- ½ Tsp. Red Pepper Flakes
- 1 Tbsp. Garlic
- 3 Tbsp. Butter, Unsalted
- Oz. Tomatoes, Canned, Diced & Undrained
- 1 Tsp. Oregano
- 1 Tsp. Sea Salt, Fine
- 1 Cup Feta Cheese, Crumbled
- ½ Cup Black Olives, Sliced
- ¼ Cup Parsley, Chopped
- 1 lb. Shrimp, Frozen & Peeled

Directions:

1. Press sauté, and then add in your butter. Once the butter begins to bubble and get foamy, add in your red pepper flakes and garlic, cooking for a minute. They should become fragrant.
2. Mix in your oregano, tomatoes, salt, and onion. Stir well, and then add your frozen shrimp.
3. Secure your lid, and then cook on low pressure for a minute. Use a quick release, and then add in your tomato broth.
4. Let this mixture to cool for a while, and then scatter olives, feta cheese and parsley over. You can serve this warm on its own or over mashed cauliflower.

Nutrition:

Calories 120

Fat 3g

Carbs 7g

Protein 15g

Roasted Chicken

Preparation Time: 10 minutes

Cooking Time: 45 minutes

Servings: 4

Ingredients:

- 2 Tbsp. Rosemary, Fresh
- 1 Tbsp. Sea Salt, Fine
- ½ Tbsp. Black Pepper
- 1 Bay leaf
- 1 Tbsp. Thyme
- 1 tbsp. Olive Oil
- 1 Chicken, Whole
- 1 Tbsp. Lemon Juice, Fresh

Directions:

1. Press sauté, and then drizzle your olive oil. Cook your chicken, flipping once before placing it to the side.

2. Add in your stand, and then add in your lemon juice, rosemary, chicken stock, and thyme. Season with salt and pepper.
3. Press poultry, and close the lid. Cook for 25 to 30 minutes.
4. Allow to cool before serving. Remember to remove your bay leaf.

Nutrition:

Calories 250

Fat 31g

Carbs 1g

Protein 30g

Salsa Chicken

Preparation Time: 5 minutes

Cooking Time: 15 minutes

Servings: 6

Ingredients:

- ½ Tsp. Chili
- 1 Tbsp. Paprika
- ½ Tbsp. Cumin
- 17 Oz. Salsa Verde
- 2 lbs. chicken Breasts, Boneless & Skinless
- 1 Tbsp. Black Pepper
- 1 Tbsp. sea Salt
- ½ Onion, Diced
- 1 Jalapeno, Diced
- ¼ Cup Cilantro, Fresh & Chopped
- 1 Lime, Fresh

Directions:

1. Put half of your salsa into the Air Fryer, and then season with salt and pepper. Add in your cilantro, jalapeno, and onion. Add in your chicken, and mix well.

2. Add in another quarter of salsa, and then place your other ¼ cup to the side. Close the lid, and cook on high heat for 10 minutes. Use a quick release, and then shred your chicken.

3. Put it back in your pot, and then add in your lime juice and salsa.

Nutrition:

Calories 96

Fat 9g

Carbs 3g

Protein 11g

Italian Shredded Chicken

Preparation Time: 5 minutes

Cooking Time: 15 minutes

Servings: 8

Ingredients:

- 1 Tbsp. Italian Seasoning
- 4 lbs. Chicken Breasts
- ½ Tsp. Sea Salt, Fine
- ½ Tsp. Ground Black Pepper
- 1 Cup Chicken Broth

Directions:

1. Lay your chicken in the Air Fryer, and then add in your seasoning. Spice it well, and then pour your broth over your chicken.
2. Cook on high pressure for 10 minutes, and then shred into strips before serving with broth.

Nutrition:

Calories 170

Fat 7g

Carbs 1g

Protein 27g

Zoodle Soup

Preparation Time: 5 minutes

Cooking Time: 25 minutes

Servings: 6

Ingredients:

- 1 Tbsp. Olive oil
- 1 Onion, Diced
- 1 lb. Chicken Breasts, Boneless, Skinless & Sliced
- 2 Cloves Garlic, Minced
- 3 Carrots, Sliced
- 1 Bay leaf
- 6 Cups Chicken Broth
- 3 Stalks Celery, Sliced
- 1 Jalapeno Pepper, Diced
- 2 Tbsp. Apple Cider Vinegar
- 4 Zucchinis, Spiralized
- Sea Salt & Black Pepper to Taste

Directions:

1. Choose sauté, and then add in your garlic and onion. Cook until you can smell the aroma, and then add in your celery, carrots, jalapeno and chicken breasts. Stir for a minute before seasoning with salt and pepper.
2. Mix in your bay leaf, chicken broth, and apple cider vinegar. Close the lid, and cook on high pressure for 20 minutes before using a quick release.
3. Choose sauté again, and then add in your zucchini, cooking for another three minutes. Serve warm.

Nutrition:

Calories 164

Fat 5g

Carbs 10g

Protein 19g

Cabbage Soup

Preparation Time: 10 minutes

Cooking Time: 35 minutes

Servings: 6

Ingredients:

- 1 Onion, Chopped
- 1 Tbsp. Avocado Oil
- 1 lb. Ground Beef
- ½ Tsp. Garlic Powder
- 1 Can Tomatoes, diced
- Sea Salt & Black Pepper to Taste
- 6 Cups Bone Broth
- 1 lb. Cabbage, Shredded
- 2 Bay Leaves

Directions:

1. Choose sauté, and then add in your oil. Once it heats up, sauté your beef and onions. Flavor with garlic, salt and pepper. Cook for 2 minutes, and then add in your bone broth, , cabbage, bay leaves and diced tomatoes.
2. Cook on high pressure for thirty minutes.
3. Use a quick release, and serve warm.

Nutrition:

Calories 428

Fat 24.8g

Carbs 9.2g

Protein 26.3g

Mojo Chicken

Preparation Time: 10 minutes

Cooking Time: 45 minutes

Servings: 4

Ingredients:

- 1 Tbsp. Lemon Juice, Fresh
- 1 Tbsp. Olive oil
- 1 Whole chicken
- 2 Tbsp. Rosemary, Fresh & Chopped
- 1 Tbsp., Fresh & Chopped
- Sea Salt & Black Pepper to Taste
- 1 Bay Leaf

Directions:

1. Choose sauté, and then add in your olive oil. Mix in your chicken, and sauté on both sides. Set aside, and then add in your trivet.

2. Mix in your lemon juice, chicken stock, rosemary and thyme. Flavor with salt and pepper, and then press your poultry button.
3. Cook for 25-30 mins., and then remove the bay leaf before serving.

Nutrition:

Calories 250

Fat 31g

Carbs 1g

Protein 30g

Spiced Almonds

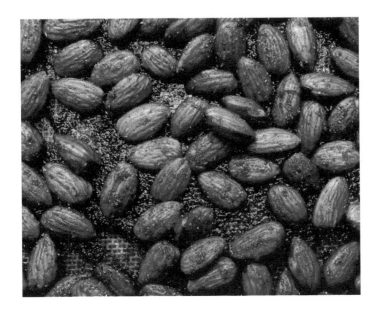

Preparation Time: 5 minutes

Cooking time: 12 minutes

Servings: 4

Ingredients:

- ½ tsp. ground cinnamon
- ½ tsp. smoked paprika

- 1 cup almonds
- 1 egg white
- Sea salt to taste

Directions:

1. Preheat Air Fryer to 310°F. Grease the Air Fryer basket with cooking spray. In a bowl, beat the egg white with cinnamon and paprika and stir in almonds.
2. Spread the almonds on the bottom of the frying basket and Air Fry for 12 minutes, shaking once or twice. Remove and sprinkle with sea salt to serve.

Nutrition:

Calories 90

Fat 2g

Carbs 3g

Protein 5g

Crispy Cauliflower Bites

Preparation Time: 5 minutes

Cooking time: 15 minutes

Servings: 4

Ingredients:

- 1 tbsp. Italian seasoning
- 1 cup flour
- 1 cup milk
- 1 egg, beaten
- 1 head cauliflower, cut into florets

Directions

1. Preheat Air Fryer to 390°F. Grease the Air Fryer basket with cooking spray. In a bowl, mix the flour, milk, egg, and Italian seasoning. Coat the cauliflower in the mixture and drain the excess liquid.
2. Place the florets in the frying basket, spray them with cooking spray, and Air Fry for 7 minutes. Shake and

continue cooking for another 5 minutes. Allow to cool before serving.

Nutrition:

Calories 70

Fat 1g

Carbs 2g

Protein 3g

Roasted Coconut Carrots

Preparation Time: 5 minutes

Cooking time: 10 minutes

Servings: 4

Ingredients:

- 1 tbsp. coconut oil, melted
- 1 lb. horse carrots, sliced
- Salt and black pepper to taste
- ½ tsp. chili powder

Directions:

1. Preheat Air Fryer to 400°F.
2. In a bowl, mix the carrots with coconut oil, chili powder, salt, and pepper. Place in the Air Fryer and Air Fry for 7 minutes. Shake the basket and cook for another 5 minutes until golden brown. Serve.

Nutrition:

Calories 80

Fat 1g

Carbs 3g

Protein 4g

Lightning Source UK Ltd.
Milton Keynes UK
UKHW020814180621
385734UK00005B/80